$6 12

BREASTFEEDING

YOUR PRICELESS GIFT
TO YOUR BABY AND YOURSELF

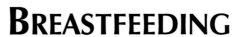

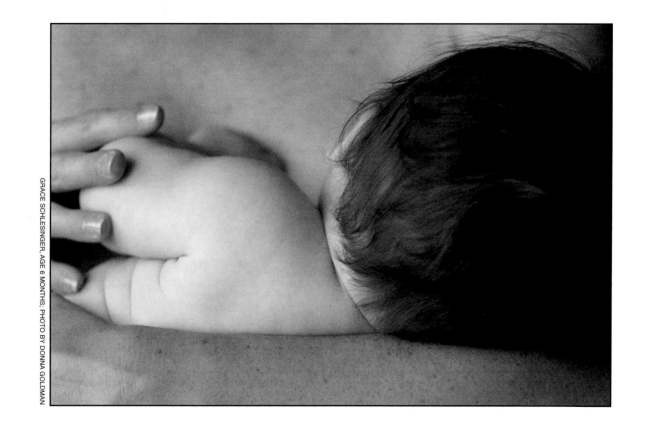

BREASTFEEDING

YOUR PRICELESS GIFT
TO YOUR BABY AND YOURSELF

Regina Sara Ryan
and
Deborah Auletta, RN, CLE
Medical Advisor: Denise Punger, MD, FAAFP, IBCLC

Hohm Press
Prescott, Arizona

Cover design: Kim Johansen
Design: Patricia Ryan
Layout: Tori Bushert

Library of Congress Cataloging in Publication Data:

Ryan, Regina Sara.
   Breastfeeding : your priceless gift to your baby and yourself / Regina Sara Ryan
   and Deborah Auletta.
      p. cm.
   ISBN 1-890772-48-8 (pbk. : alk. paper)
1. Breastfeeding—Health aspects—Popular works. I. Auletta, Deborah. II. Title.
   RJ216R936 2005
   649'.33—dc22

                                    2005005380

HOHM PRESS
P.O. Box 2501
Prescott, AZ 86302
800-381-2700
http://www.hohmpress.com

This book was printed in the U.S.A. on acid-free paper using soy ink.

09 08 07 06 05   5 4 3 2

Cover image: Five nursing mothers—Kathy Hughes, Karen Zirger, Deedee Olsen, Shayla Townsend and Belinda Holmes.
   Photographer: Denise Punger, MD

To Lee Lozowick
whose dedication to the genuine needs of all children
inspired us and gave us the courage to present this book.

ACKNOWLEDGEMENTS

Our gratitude to all the moms, dads, doctors, nurses, midwives, doulas, photographers, WIC agency representatives, friends, family and sangha members without whose generous help this book would not have happened. Thank you to Yusef for providing direct life experience.

Our appreciation to the staff at Hohm Press, Bala Zuccarello, Dasya Zuccarello and Thom Shelby for their encouragement and help, and to Elyse April, whose research assistance and overall support were invaluable to the project.

Special thanks to Denise Punger, M.D., family physician, international board certified lactation consultant and photographer, whose medical expertise and friendly advice were consistently available.

PREFACE

Most of us have an idea about how important nutrition is for overall health. High fiber, low fat, fresh fruits and vegetables, less red meat, less sugar…all promise to improve health and help prevent disease. "You are what you eat," the saying goes, and in some approaches to medicine, like traditional Chinese, diet is used as the first line of defense against illness. In contrast, a recent U.S. movie called *Supersize Me* documented what happened to a healthy guy who decided to eat only McDonald's fast food for an entire month. The effects of his little experiment to his overall health were so devastating that it prompted McDonald's to drop its "Would you like me to supersize that?" query in its marketing.

Just as what *you* eat is crucial to your health and well-being, what you decide to feed your newborn child will set the foundation for his or her health for their entire lifetime. Regina and I wrote this book because we want to support the practice of breastfeeding by sharing the most vital nutrition and health information that many moms-to-be may not be fully aware of. Although the American Academy of Pediatrics recommends breast-feeding for at least twelve months, less than twenty percent of babies in the U.S. are still nursing at this young age. How could this be, when there is so much irrefutable evidence showing that breast is best? For one thing, if your mother is of my age, of the baby boomer generation, she was probably discouraged from breastfeeding and it is likely that you were not breastfed. Only since the 1970s have the virtues of breastfeeding, which have been instinctively known for thousands of years, been scientifically studied, yielding a massive amount of information about the physical, emotional, and intellectual benefits of breastfeeding to both mom and baby. Secondly, just as McDonald's spends millions of dollars persuading the consumer to eat what's on their menu, the huge companies that produce infant formula have multimillion-dollar budgets to persuade you of the ease and health value of their products. Even with overwhelming scientific data to the contrary, breast-feeding advocates cannot compete with that kind of budget. We have had to use another approach. One to one.

Regina and I believe that, with the right information, most of you as parents will decide that breastfeeding is right for your baby. After making the decision to nurse your baby, all you need is some help and a bit of perseverance, and soon breastfeeding can be as easy as any activity of life that once seemed challenging but is now performed with ease and grace. I know this from professional and personal experience. Every day, in the Family Birthing Center at Yavapai Regional Medical Center in Prescott, Arizona, I watch nurses gently help new moms and babies begin the simple yet profound experience of breastfeeding.

Over twenty years ago my own son started his life in the Newborn Intensive Care Unit at the University of New Mexico Hospital. For more than two weeks he received no food by mouth, only intravenous fluids. Fortunately, the excellent nursing staff heard me when I said I wanted to breastfeed my baby. For that, I remain forever grateful to them. They taught me what I needed to know to protect my milk supply until my son could eat. At seventeen days of age my son nursed for the first time, and I learned that if a woman wants to breastfeed her child, she probably can.

The beginning of my son's life was so difficult—in his first four months he underwent several hospitalizations. Holding him in my arms and nursing was all that I could offer that was always a comfort to him. I believe it was a lifeline for both of us; a way for us to reconnect to one another. Although our attempts to have a normal life kept getting interrupted, breastfeeding brought us back together in a way that ultimately re-strengthened the bond between us. Even after surgery, breastfeeding provided him a way back into his young life, and to me, that was irreplaceable.

Regina and I wrote this book to empower your courage and inspiration to make the best decision for you and your baby. We hope you make the decision that thousands of women all around the world make every day—to breastfeed. *Breastfeeding: Your Priceless Gift to Your Baby and Yourself* presents you with twenty of the most compelling reasons why breast is best and why the choice to breastfeed may be one of the most important decisions you ever make as a parent.

—*Deborah Auletta*

20 REASONS IN SUPPORT OF BREASTFEEDING

"BREASTFEEDING IS THE #1 OPTION"
SAY U.S. PEDIATRICIANS AND INFANT-HEALTH AUTHORITIES AROUND THE WORLD

YOU CAN FEEL CONFIDANT THAT A DECISION TO BREASTFEED is both encouraged and supported by doctors, infant care experts and health service agencies worldwide. Pediatricians throughout the U.S., especially the American Academy of Pediatrics (A.A.P.), are clear that breastfeeding is the best option for infant feeding:

> Human milk is species-specific, and all substitute feeding preparations differ markedly from it, making human milk uniquely superior for infant feeding…Exclusive breastfeeding is sufficient to support optimal growth and development for approximately the first 6 months of life…Breastfeeding should be continued for at least the first year of life and beyond for as long as mutually desired…There is no upper limit to the duration…and no evidence of psychologic or developmental harm from breastfeeding into the third year of life or longer. —A.A.P., *Breastfeeding Policy Statement, 2005*

In the U.S., this stand is reinforced by the Surgeon General's Office, and the WIC (Women, Infants and Children) programs of the Department of Health and Human Services. The government's "Healthy People 2010" initiative aims for a 75% breastfeeding rate among all U.S. mothers by the year 2010.

Around the globe, the World Health Organization (WHO) has set standards to help educate everyone about the need for better infant health through breastfeeding. And don't forget that UNICEF (United Nations Children's Fund) calls breastfeeding "the best start to life."

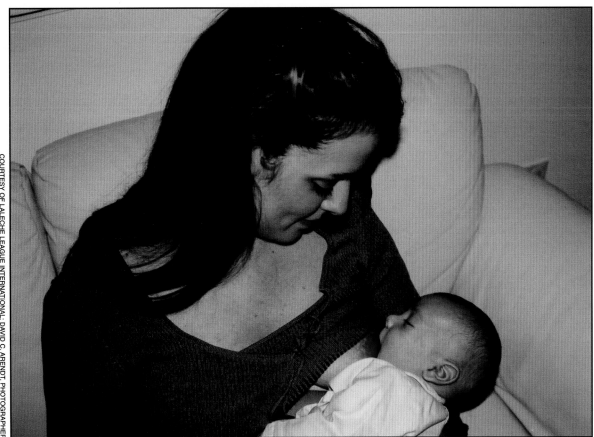

BREASTMILK IS BABY'S "PERSONALLY-DESIGNED"
AND PERFECT FOOD

THE HUMAN BODY IS AMAZING! The components of your breastmilk will change according to your baby's age and need. Even premature or sick babies will get a higher protein-content milk, naturally, through mother's body.

In their first breastfeedings, babies will receive *colostrum*—that miraculous substance that supplies many of the antibodies babies need to resist disease. Because it is rich in nutrients, only a small amount is needed, which is perfect because the newborn's stomach is the size of a walnut. Colostrum acts as a natural laxative to encourage baby's first bowel movement, which helps to avoid jaundice.

Breastmilk's nutritional balance is exact: just the right amount of fat (fatty acids), sugar (lactose), protein (amino acids), and water to assure growth and development of your baby's body. And, breastmilk uniquely nourishes the baby's brain. No infant formula can reproduce this personally-designed recipe.

The human digestive system is structured to process human milk…not cow's-milk-based formula, or cow's milk, the main component of most formulas, which has much larger protein molecules, and may contain growth hormones that unnaturally encourage weight gain…and not soy-based formulas, which may produce allergic reactions.

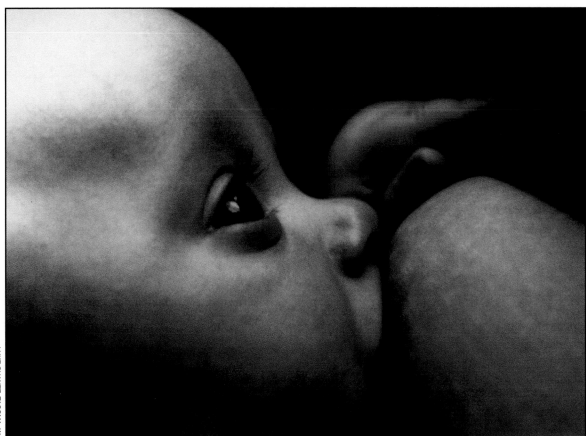

ALLERGIES AND ASTHMA ARE LESS LIKELY
WITH BREASTFEEDING

WHILE ALLERGIES AMONG CHILDREN IN GENERAL HAVE INCREASED ENORMOUSLY in the last twenty years, statistics compiled by La Leche League International show that breastfed babies are seven times less likely to get them.

Allergies and asthma tend to run in a family, sometimes for several generations back. But, breastfeeding for at least six to twelve months can help discourage that cycle. The colostrum in breastmilk will begin to "seal" your baby's intestinal lining, making a natural barrier against allergens and bacteria. Even one supplementation of cow-based formula will negatively affect this process. Since it takes at least six months for the immune system to develop, your breastmilk will help build the strongest immune system possible for your baby.

Furthermore, the longer you feed your infant only breastmilk, the more protection you offer, since the likelihood of developing an allergy to a food or substance increases the longer it is consumed. Keeping to breastmilk, you protect your child from the allergens present in cow's milk (which contains over twenty known allergy-producing substances), and soy-based milk (also an allergic substance), which are the basis of most infant formulas.

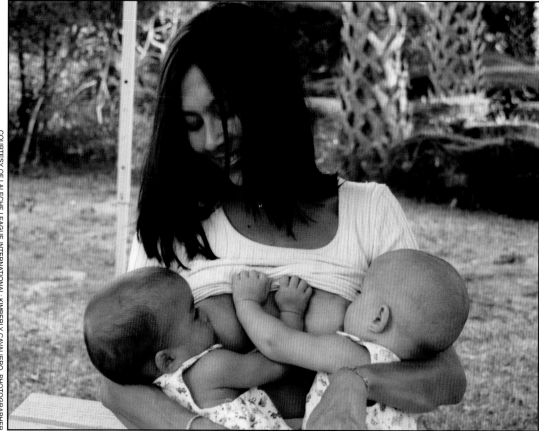

BREASTFEEDING PROTECTS BABIES FROM ILLNESS

THE HUMAN IMMUNE SYSTEM DEPENDS ON ANTIBODIES—tiny protein molecules that serve as the first line of defense against particular bacteria or viruses. As soon as a bacterial "invader" is recognized, its antibody (like an "antidote") kicks into action to round up and eliminate the threatening agent.

Antibodies that protect from a wide variety of serious diseases are passed from mother to infant through the placenta. Another large supply comes through mother's breastmilk. When babies breastfeed, they receive the optimal protection against many childhood illnesses, some of which (like leukemia and meningitis) could threaten their lives; others, like asthma and allergies, that can affect their health and well being indefinitely.

Research verifies that breastfed babies have:

> ❧ less childhood ear infections, especially those that damage hearing ❧ less digestive disorders, especially diarrhea ❧ less respiratory illnesses like pneumonia and asthma ❧ less skin problems, like eczema ❧ less childhood cancer: including leukemia and Hodgkin's disease ❧ less Crohn's disease ❧ less bacterial meningitis ❧ less diabetes ❧ less SIDS

Breastfeeding is also shown to increase the baby's visual acuity and the body's ability to use the antibodies contained in childhood vaccines.

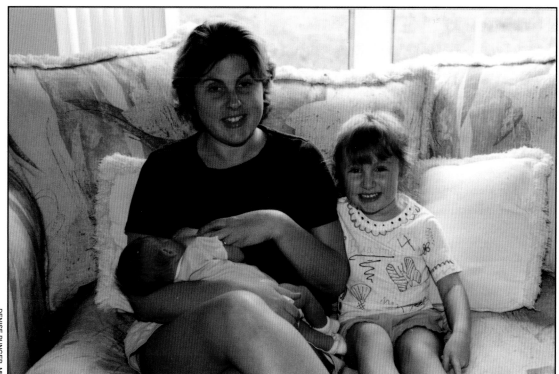

BREASTFEEDING SAVES BABIES LIVES

STATISTICS ON RATES OF INFANT MORTALITY have long been used as measures of a culture's overall level of health and development. Even in poorer nations, breastfeeding is a life saver! Breastfed infants suffer much less from diarrhea, a principle factor in the dehydration leading to death. They are also ideally protected from malnutrition and from the effects of the bacteria and viruses that threaten other infants so severely. Estimates offered by the United Nations are that 1.5 million babies' lives would be saved every year if all babies were breastfed.

Even in the U.S., infant mortality rates are decreased by breastfeeding. Regardless of their race, breastfed children between 28 days and one year of life had a 20 percent lower risk of dying, and the percentage of advantage increased the longer the child was breastfed. Separate research has shown that breastfeeding reduces the incidence of SIDS (Sudden Infant Death Syndrome).

Despite remarkable and sophisticated health services, the U.S. ranks #30 in the world for infant mortality. More widespread acceptance of breastfeeding could help change that!

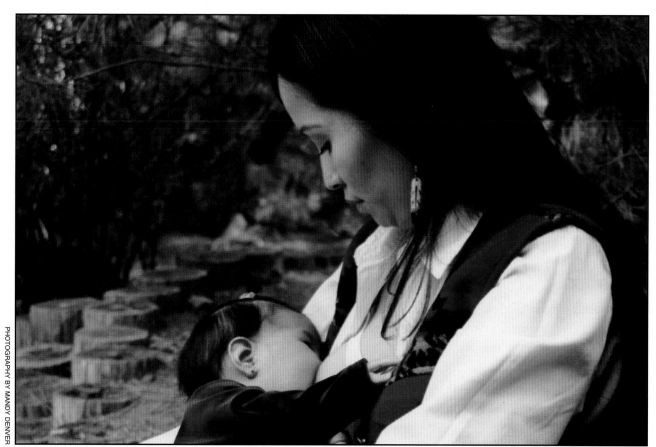

BREASTFED BABIES NEED FEWER DOCTOR VISITS

PEDIATRICIANS AND FAMILY DOCTORS TYPICALLY SEE DOZENS OF BABIES in their offices every week. Their records show that breastfed babies generally require fewer visits for sickness than formula-fed babies do. Because breastfed babies have less infections, less digestion disorders, less respiratory problems, less ear disturbances…this also adds up to fewer hospital admissions.

The connections multiply when you consider that less sickness for baby means that parents don't have to take off as much time from work or home care, or just plain fun, to bring their child to a doctor or to stay with their child in a hospital. Less illness naturally means that the family is spending less money on medicines or services, money that can be used for other things.

Time and money saved is only a part of the picture, however. Fewer doctor visits mean much less anxiety and stress for both parents and child. It isn't just a physical body that gets sick. Any child's illness adds to the overall emotional tension and worry that parents normally have to bear. Breastfeeding supports the wellness of body, mind and spirit for the whole family.

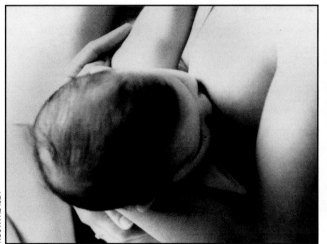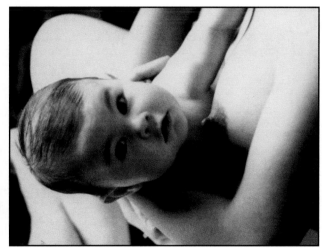

Breastmilk Feeds the Brain...
and Links to Increased Intelligence

CHILDREN WHO WERE FED HUMAN BREASTMILK EXCLUSIVELY for the first 6 months of life, despite their mothers' education or social background, were found to have better motor skills and higher intelligence scores than those who were fed infant formula or both breastmilk and other food sources.

Several important studies have confirmed these same findings. As measured by both infant-development scales and later IQ tests, breastfed children scored an average 10 points higher than formula-fed children at age 7-8.

Groundbreaking research at the National Institute of Child Health and Human Development (NICHD) recently found that two amino acids present only in breastmilk are responsible for stimulating the infant's brain: "This study provides strong evidence that exclusive breastfeeding for the first six months benefits the cognitive development of both small and normal-size infants. Also...breastfeeding does not compromise growth," said Duane Alexander, M.D., Director of the NICHD.

Other experts assert that breastmilk nourishes the part of the brain responsible for motor skills, and all these benefits are maximized when a child nurses for two years or longer.

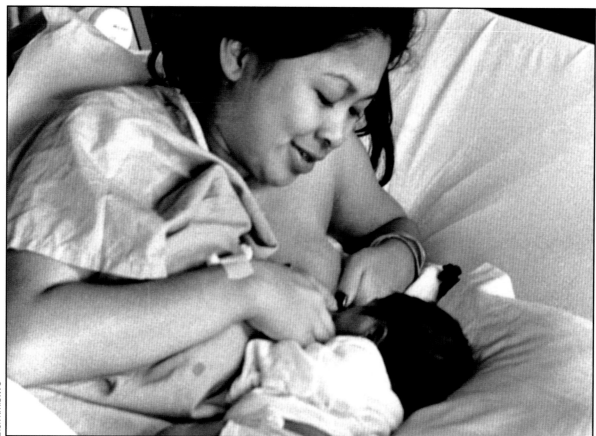

PHYSICAL/EMOTIONAL BONDING BETWEEN
MOTHER AND CHILD IS INCREASED BY BREASTFEEDING

THE MOTHER-INFANT BOND IS PROBABLY THE STRONGEST RELATIONSHIP that exists in the world. From the baby's perspective, bonding with mother is a matter of life or death!

Babies experience anxiety when they are separated from human contact, or when their food is lacking. Having these needs met quickly and consistently, babies relax and learn to trust…which at this stage equates to *love*. It is extremely difficult to measure the strength of the bond between any individual baby and mother because so many factors are at play. However, breastfed babies generally get more skin-to-skin contact and more stroking than bottle-fed infants do. And skin contact and stroking have been shown to affect a child significantly. When premature babies, for instance, are nestled skin-to-skin against the mother's chest, kangaroo-style, they grow and gain weight more quickly. This also helps them develop a regular heartbeat and breathing pattern—which literally saves their lives.

Breastfed infants also establish more constant eye contact with mother, a factor that increases the bonding. Many believe that the failure to affectionately bond in the first years of life is responsible for many disease-related conditions and social and behavioral problems in both children and adults later in life.

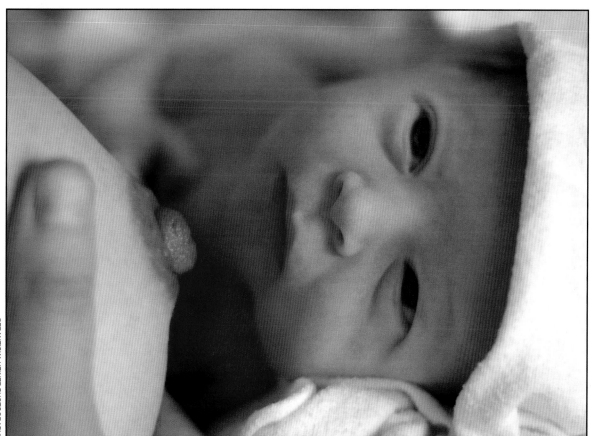

BREASTFED BABIES HAVE LESS NEED TO CRY

ALL BABIES CRY—IT IS A NORMAL PART OF THEIR DEVELOPMENT, and one of their earliest forms of communication. Babies have needs: for food, for feeling safe, for relief from pain or discomfort…Crying alerts us that something needs our attention.

Some babies cry less than others, however. Babies whose needs are met quickly and consistently cry less in the first year than babies whose needs are not quickly met. And, research shows that breastfed babies don't cry as much overall as bottle-fed babies. Most breastfed babies have less colic, a big reason for crying, and since they don't have to wait for formula or bottle fixings, they aren't crying from hunger.

Wherever you are, day or night, your breastfed baby is usually only a moment away from the nurturance of your milk, plus the exquisite comfort of contact with your skin. Your breastmilk contains endorphins—natural substances that help in decreasing pain and promoting relaxation leading to sleep. So, whether your child is hungry, or emotionally upset, breastfeeding can help soothe the hurt. That can mean less crying for your infant and more ease and confidence for you.

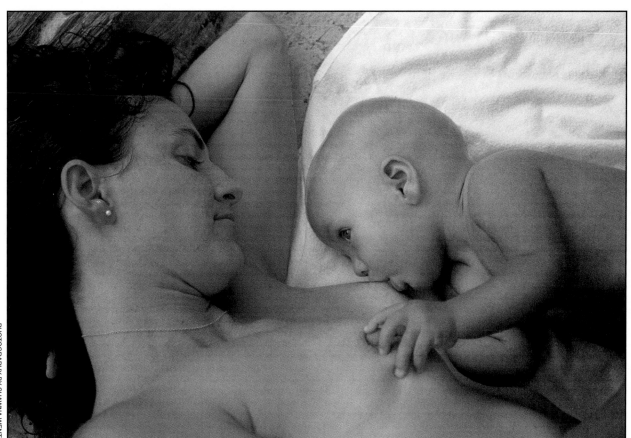

BREASTFEEDING ENCOURAGES STRESS REDUCTION
IN BABY AND MOM

THE PACE OF OUR MODERN LIVES, with the added responsibility for a new child, are already challenging. Mothers and babies can profit tremendously from the stress reduction that comes as a natural consequence of breastfeeding.

In the breastfeeding process, the hormone prolactin (sometimes called the "mothering hormone") promotes positive feelings in the nursing mother. It also serves as a relaxant for baby. The hormone oxytocin, which regulates milk ejection from the breast (known as "let down"), is the same one released in your body during lovemaking. As a result, strengthened feelings of closeness, love, and warmth toward your baby are the natural outcome of breastfeeding.

Stress is also lessened throughout your child's early years if he or she is healthy most of the time. Because breastfed babies require fewer doctor visits and hospital stays, family stress is reduced.

Finally, increased holding and carrying of a baby has been proven to mean less crying…and that means less stress for family and baby. Breastfeeding moms have the added advantage of more time to hold and caress their infants.

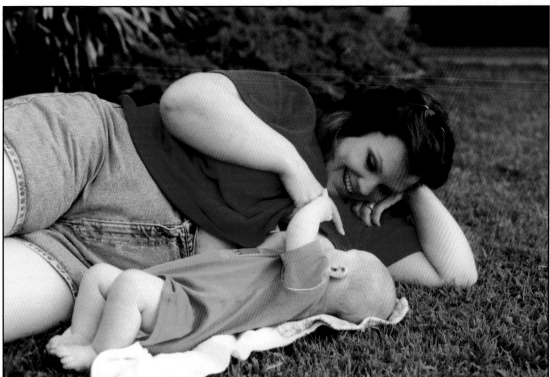

Breastfeeding Is *Much Less* Costly
than Formula Feeding

BREASTMILK IS FREE, AND IT USUALLY STAYS IN GENEROUS SUPPLY. The more your baby nurses, the more your milk production is stimulated. The reduced stress and expense of fewer doctor visits and hospital stays for breastfed babies makes breastfeeding the most economic alternative in the U.S. and in countries around the world.

As long as it is the exclusive form of infant feeding, breastfeeding will save an average U.S. family *at least* a thousand dollars annually. The cost of formula and equipment can exceed over $4000 per year, depending upon whether or not an infant is being fed special allergy-free substitutes. Even if a nursing mother needs a breastmilk pump or other items, breastfeeding is still her most economic option.

In poorer countries, the costs of formula/bottle feeding can be outrageous—sometimes representing more than the entire household's annual income. For both individuals and for nations, therefore, breastfeeding reduces overall healthcare spending.

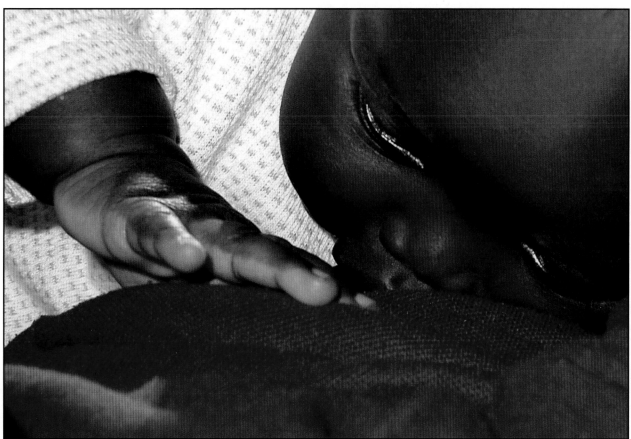

BREASTFEEDING BUILDS STRAIGHTER TEETH
AND STRONGER TEETH

TEETH START TO FORM UNDER THE GUMS EVEN BEFORE A CHILD A BORN. Therefore, how your baby nurses (either from breast or bottle) will affect the way the primary teeth ("baby teeth") grow in…setting the stage for permanent teeth.

Research in 2004 indicated that a baby who gets food and comfort from sucking the breast is ***twice as likely*** to have better-positioned teeth than those who are fed with a rubberized bottle-nipple, or "comforted" with a substitute pacifier. Experts in both dentistry and childhood disease believe that how these primary or "baby" teeth are positioned and spaced can be crucial for correct jaw alignment and positioning as permanent teeth eventually start to grow in.

Other tooth-related advantages of breastfeeding are that suckling helps to build the ideal mouth structure that can decrease speech impediments and the need for orthodontics (braces) in later years. Also, when bottles are propped up next to the baby, this practice may lead to tooth decay because formula tends to pool in the babies mouth during sleep.

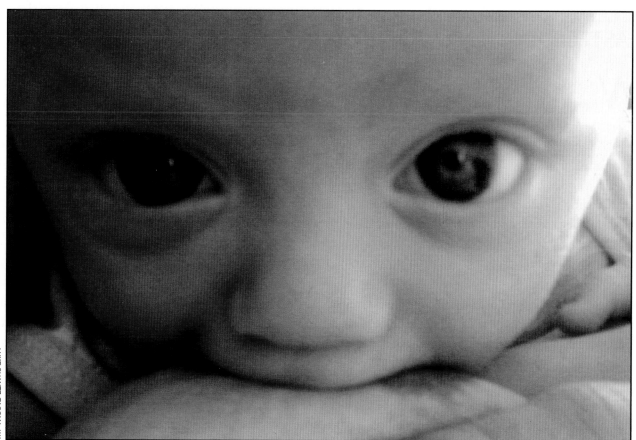

BREASTFEEDING IS GOOD FOR THE EARTH

WHEN YOU ACTUALLY START TO LIST ALL THE WAYS that formula/bottle feeding affects the planet, the implications multiply. Just think of all the packaging material that gets used in formula presentation, and all the glass, plastic and rubber that gets manufactured for bottles and nipples and substitutes. Consider the resources used in advertising these products and the energy you would spend in shopping for them, storing them, heating them, washing or sterilizing them, replacing them, and disposing of them.

Breastfeeding is "eco-efficient"—which means that breastfeeding encourages the use of naturally-existing technologies (the human body's own energy sources) rather than depleting the earth's resources or depending on manufactured products that may themselves be contaminated and that lead to increased pollution.

In poorer countries, these factors are especially damaging to the environment, especially where water is scarce. Nearly four extra quarts of water a day—some for mixing in formula and the rest for sterilizing bottles—may be needed. When wood fires are used to boil water, this adds an additional burden on the environment and on the family, typically to the mother herself who is generally responsible for gathering or cutting wood and collecting or carrying water.

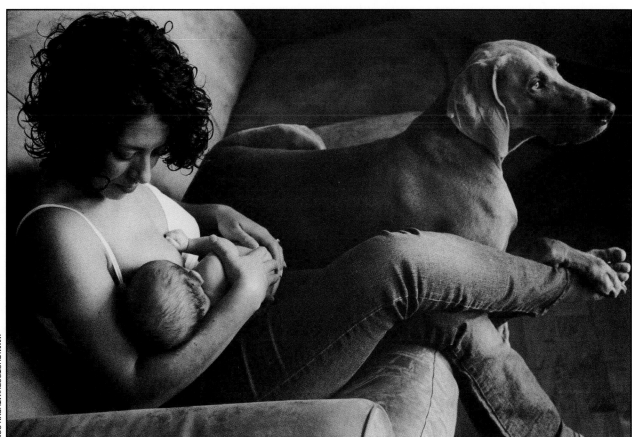

BREASTFEEDING HELPS MOTHER'S BODY READJUST
AFTER PREGNANCY

OBVIOUSLY PREGNANCY WILL CHANGE (or has changed) a lot of things in your body, as well as in your mind. Your weight, the size of your uterus, your emotional sensitivity, your outlook on life…all are affected by the presence of new life in your womb. You know it!

What you may not know is that, by breastfeeding your infant, these body-mind changes that occur during pregnancy are balanced out and taken care of very specifically by your body's natural wisdom. Breastfeeding encourages normal readjustment once your baby has arrived. Breastfeeding can be emotionally healing for a negative birth experience.

The key to this readjustment is the hormone oxytocin. As soon as your baby latches onto your breast and begins suckling repeatedly, oxytocin starts releasing from your pituitary gland. This oxytocin signals the breast to start releasing milk. At the same time, however, oxytocin starts contractions in the uterus. This necessary function protects the uterus from possible hemorrhage and encourages its return to its original size. Without breastfeeding, the uterus does not fully return to pre-pregnancy size.

Because breastmilk-production uses up 200-500 extra calories per day, breastfeeding moms will find it easier to lose the extra weight gained during pregnancy.

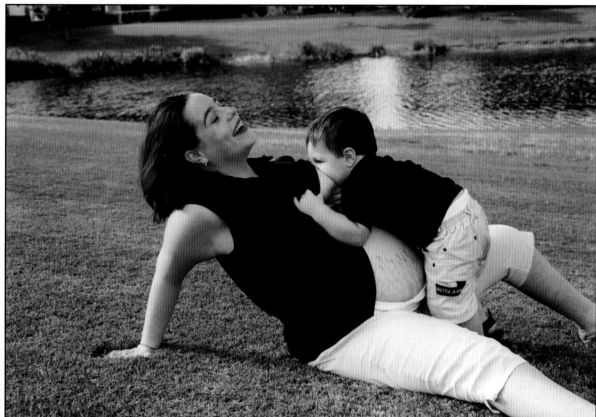

BREASTFEEDING ALSO PROTECTS A MOTHER'S HEALTH...
THROUGHOUT HER LIFE

CURRENT RESEARCH IS FOCUSING MORE AND MORE on the incomparable health advantages to mothers who breastfeed their babies—advantages that magnify the longer a woman breastfeeds. Besides the remarkable immediate benefits—like easier weight-loss and less risk of hemorrhage or anemia following birth—the effects on a mother's long-term health are astounding medical practitioners everywhere.

Studies now indicate that women who have breastfed their children may have:

    ❧ less breast cancer ❧ less ovarian cancer ❧ less endometriosis ❧ less osteoporosis ❧ less insulin requirements (in diabetic women) ❧ less risk of heart problems ❧ less risk of rheumatoid arthritis

The "why" behind this natural protection is still under investigation. In some cases, credit is being given to the way that breastfeeding helps to regulate the usage of estrogen in the body, an advantage that non-breast-feeding mothers do not share.

One thing is certain: the initial findings are important enough that the subject has captured the attention of medical researchers throughout the world.

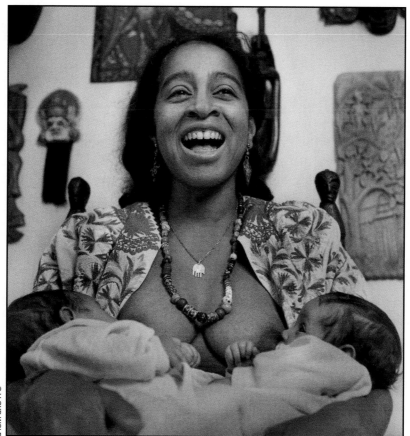

BREASTFEEDING BUILDS A WOMAN'S SELF-CONFIDENCE

BECOMING A MOTHER CERTAINLY TRANSFORMS A WOMAN'S LIFE. When mother breastfeeds, these positive transformations increase.

Feeding your child from your own body makes *you* the center of your child's life. Knowing how important this unique nourishment is, and how many priceless advantages you are giving your newborn, your self-esteem will naturally grow. Learning the wonders of your body, and living in tune with its rhythms and the rhythms of your baby's body, you will naturally develop a greater sense of body-trust, which is one factor that builds your self-confidence.

In a remarkable survey study done in Kentucky (1984) among women participating in WIC services, mothers who breastfed reported more self-esteem and assertiveness than mothers who had not. They also interacted more maturely with their infants. As time went by, the nursing moms turned their lives around by going back to school in greater numbers than their non-breastfeeding peers. They got jobs and provided more adequately for their infants.

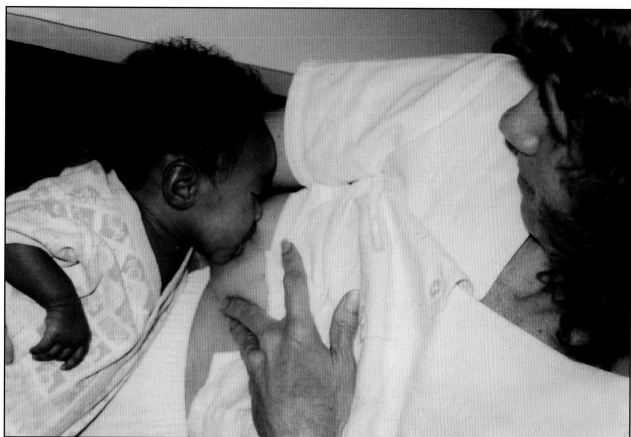

BREASTFEEDING HONORS A WOMAN'S BODY

"BEFORE I HAD MY BABY I ONLY THOUGHT ABOUT my breasts as being sexy or not...or as making me look good or not." Connie, a young mother, shared her experience as she breastfed her three-month-old infant girl.

"Now, I appreciate my breasts in a whole new way. They are a 'mama's breasts,' they carry 'mama's milk.' I love the fact that I am feeding my baby from my own body. Breastfeeding has helped me *so much* to let go of my fears and comparisons about my body, especially about my breasts."

Women's breasts *are* considered sexy in our culture, but often this view becomes distorted and limited. Breasts are so much more than "sex objects." For Connie, breastfeeding her child became a sacred and womanly art—an expression of a mother's participation in nature's design for human life. As a breastfeeding mother, she felt herself connected to women throughout the world, and to generations of women before her. Breastfeeding has helped Connie and many other women to trust and honor their bodies.

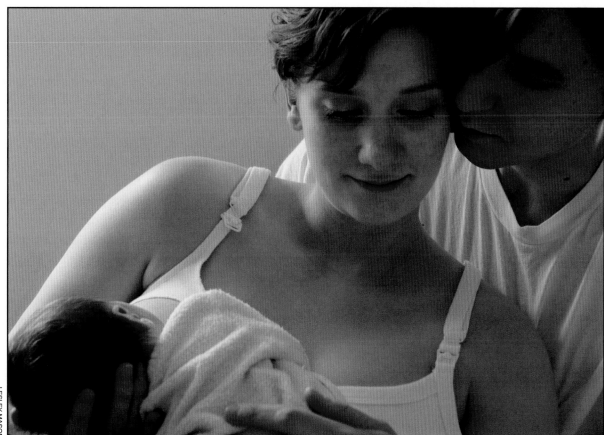

BREASTFEEDING MAKES TRAVEL EASIER

WHETHER YOU ARE DRIVING TO THE MALL TO SHOP, or flying cross-country to visit relatives or friends, breastfeeding means that your baby's food supply is never in question. That one "small" detail in travel can make a huge difference. You don't have to pack or carry anything special. You don't have to delay feeding unnecessarily while bottles or formulas are prepared and heated. You don't have to rely on shopping for supplies, using water, or cleaning up in a new environment. Summer or winter, your breastmilk is always the right temperature for your baby to immediately take. Whether you are eating your normal diet or trying out the cuisine of a new place, your breastmilk will still provide your baby with the perfect balance of nutrients.

Travel can sometimes be stressful on baby, especially if it is stressful for you. But, the natural sedative-like hormones in breastmilk and those released in your body when you breastfeed (like prolactin) will help encourage relaxation in both of you.

The African word "Mamatoto" says it well—"mama" (mother) and "toto" (baby) are bonded. They go everywhere together. The two now travel as one.

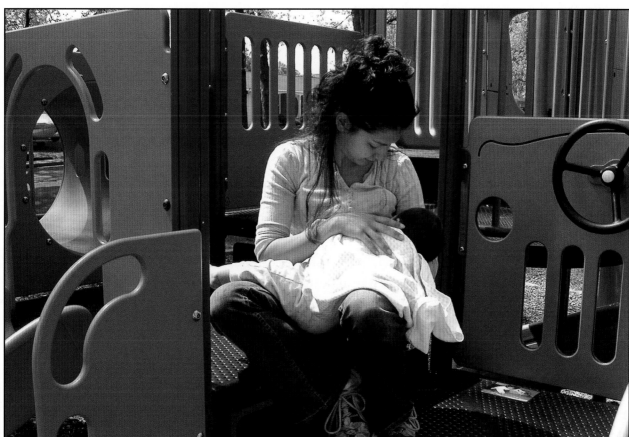

Breastfed Babies Smell Better

IF YOU'VE EVER SMELLED AND/OR TASTED INFANT FORMULAS you probably appreciate this point without question. These products can vary in taste and consistency from thick and pasty, to sour, to watery and medicinal. Breastmilk, by contrast, is naturally sweet, and light. It doesn't stain your clothes or baby's clothes, while formulas typically leave a stain that is difficult to remove.

Although all babies will spit up, since breastmilk is so much more digestible, babies who breastfeed will normally spit up less. With the smaller, frequent feedings that breastfeeding encourages, breastmilk is digested faster in the stomach, and is ready to be absorbed by the rest of the body.

If breastmilk is regurgitated, however, it rarely smells offensive, and doesn't leave a stale, sour residue on baby's clothing, in baby's hair or on baby's skin, the way milk-substitutes do. Baby's bowel movements are less strong-smelling when they are breastfed as opposed to the poops of bottle-fed babies, which can be quite powerful.

All together, breastfed babies will typically smell better, sweeter, and more natural…more of the time. No small factor for busy mothers, and for those who take their infants everywhere.

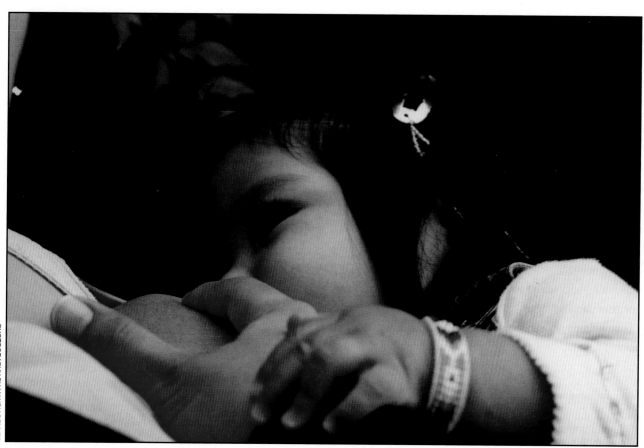

BREASTFEEDING IS NATURE'S OBVIOUS PLAN

THE MOTHER'S BREAST IS DESIGNED TO FEED AND NURTURE the newborn of the human species, and babies know this, instinctively! Without assistance, a newborn that is placed on mother's abdomen will crawl to her breast, find her nipple, latch on and begin to suckle.

Yet, in modern times, starting in the early 1900s, many of our mothers and grandmothers were convinced by irresponsible infant-formula manufacturers, and other ill-advised "experts" and friends, that bottle-feeding was "the better way—the modern way." In the process of accepting this, however, they had to deny the obvious by replacing breastfeeding with a plastic bottle filled with re-constituted infant formula.

The knowledge of "nature's way" is universal. While people may not choose to follow the obvious, everybody who looks can see how the human body is structured. If we, women, stop long enough to listen to what our feminine bodily wisdom is saying to us, we will understand that mother's milk is intended as baby's first food. It is baby's right and privilege to be breastfed.

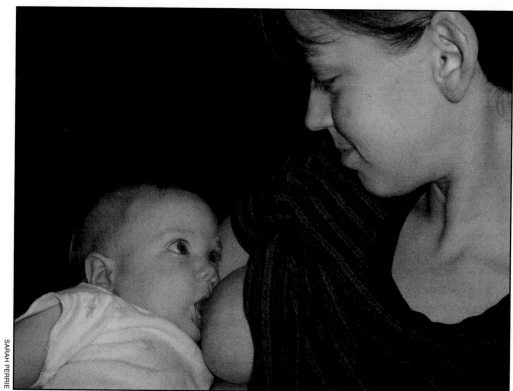

GENERAL REFERENCES

Lawrence, R.A., and R.M. Lawrence, *Breastfeeding: A Guide for the Medical Profession*, 5th Edition, St. Louis, Missouri: Mosby, 1999.

Mohrbacher, N., and J. Stock, *La Leche League International, The Breastfeeding Answer Book*, 3rd revised edition, Schaumburg, Illinois: La Leche League International, 2003. *Also see:* www.lalecheleague.org

Sears, W. and M. Sears, *The Baby Book: Everything You Need to Know About Your Baby from Birth to Age Two* (revised and updated edition), New York: Little, Brown and Company, 2003.

Sears, W. and M. Sears, *The Breastfeeding Book*, New York: Little, Brown & Co., 2000.

REFERENCES TO INDIVIDUAL REASONS

REASON 1: "BREASTFEEDING IS THE #1 OPTION," SAY U.S. PEDIATRICIANS AND INFANT-HEALTH AUTHORITIES FROM AROUND THE WORLD

The A.A.P. Policy Statement "Breastfeeding and the Use of Human Milk (1 Feb. 2005) can be viewed at:
http://aappolicy.aappublications.org/cgi/content/full/pediatrics;115/2/496

"Healthy People 2010," U.S. Goals for health as issued by Centers for Disease Control and Prevention Health Resources and Services Administration. To find items relating to breastfeeding go to: http://www.healthypeople.gov/Search/objectives/htm
Search by keyword: breastfeeding

UNICEF Publication, *Breastfeeding: Foundation for a Healthy Future*, August 1999. www.unicef.org

REASON 2: BREASTMILK IS BABY'S "PERSONALLY-DESIGNED" AND PERFECT FOOD

Jensen, R.G. (editor) *Handbook of Milk Composition*, San Diego, Calif: Academic Press, 1995.

See: http://www.askdrsears.com/html/2/T021600.asp
"Comparison Chart of Breastfeeding vs. Formula Feeding Regarding the composition of Human Breastmilk"

REASON 3: ASTHMA AND ALLERGIES ARE LESS LIKELY WITH BREASTFEEDING

See: http://allergies.about.com/cs/breastfeeding/a/aa073100a.htm
A study in the December 1999 issue of the *Journal of Allergy and Clinical Immunology* showed that colostrum may help prevent the development of inherited allergies. Colostrum is high in protein and antibodies. During the study it appeared it also promoted antibody production.

See: http://allergies.about.com/library/blaaaai072202a.htm
A study in the July 2002 issue of the *Journal of Allergy and Clinical Immunology* found that exclusively breast feeding infants for at least four months provided them protection from developing asthma.

REASON 4: BREASTFEEDING PROTECTS BABIES FROM ILLNESS

Beaudry, M., R. Dufour and S. Marcoux, "Relation Between Infant Feeding and Infections During the First 6 Months of Life." *Journal of Pediatrics* 126:191-197, 1995. PubMed; PMID 7844664

Birch, E., D. Birch and D. Hoffman, et.al.: "Breastfeeding and Optimal Visual Development," *Journal of Pediatr Ophthalmol Strabismus*, 30:33, 1993.

Davis, M.K., "Review of the Evidence for an Association Between Infant Feeding and Childhood Cancer." In: International Union Against Cancer (UICC, WHO) Workshop: "Nutritional morbidity in children with cancer: mechanisms, measures, and management." *Int J Cancer Suppl.* 1998,11:29-33.

REFERENCES

Duncan, B., J. Ey and C.J. Holberg, et al., "Exclusive Breast-Feeding for at Least 4 Months Protects Against Otitis Media." *Pediatrics,* 91:867-872, 1993. PubMed; PMID 8474804

Frank, A.L., L.H. Taber and W.P. Glezen, et al. "Breast-feeding and Respiratory Virus Infection." *Pediatrics,* 70:239-245, 1982. PubMed; PMID 7099789

Howell, R.R., R.H. Morriss, Jr., L.D. Pickering, editors, *Human Milk in Infant Nutrition and Health*, Springfield, Ill.: Thomas Publishers, 1986.

Howie, P.W., J.S. Forsyth and S.A. Ogston, et al. "Protective Effect of Breast Feeding Against Infection." *British Medical Journal* 300:11-16, 1990. PubMed; PMID 2105113

Kovar, M.G., M.K. Serdula and J.S. Marks, et al. "Review of the Epidemiologic Evidence for An Association between Infant Feeding and Infant Health." *Pediatrics,* 74:S615-S638, 1984. PubMed; PMID 6384916

Saarinen, U.M., "Prolonged breast feeding as prophylaxis for recurrent otitis media." *Acta Paediatric Scandinavica* 71:567-571, 1982. PubMed; PMID 7136672

Slusser, W., M.D., Director, UCLA Breastfeeding Resource Program, "Medical Advantages of Breastfeeding," presentation at the UCLA Lactation Education Program, Long Beach, California, 2004.

Telemo, E. and L.A. Hanson, "Antibodies in Milk," *Journal of Mammary Gland Biol. Neoplasia*, 1:243, 1996.

Wright, A.L., C.J. Holberg and L.M. Taussig, et al. "Relationship of Infant Feeding to Recurrent Wheezing at Age 6 Years." *Archives of Pediatric and Adolescent Medicine,* 149:758-763, 1995. PubMed; PMID 7795765

Xiao, O. S. and M. S. Linet, et al., "Breast-Feeding and Risk of Childhood Acute Leukemia," *Journal of the National Cancer Institute*, Vol. 91, No. 20, 1765-1772, October 20, 1999.

REASON 5: BREASTFEEDING SAVES BABIES LIVES

Cunningham, A.S., D.B. Jelliffe, and E.R.P. Jelliffe, "Breastfeeding and Health in the 1980's: A Global Epidemiologic Review," *Journal of Pediatrics*, 118: 659, 1991.

Oyen, N., et. al., "Combined Effects of Sleeping Position and Prenatal Risk Factors in Sudden Infant Death Syndrome: The Nordic Epidemiological SIDS," *Pediatrics*, Vol. 100 No. 4 October 1997, 613-621.

Popkin, B.M.; Adair, L.; Akin, J.S.; et al. "Breast-feeding and Diarrheal Morbidity." *Pediatrics* 86:874-882, 1990. PubMed; PMID 2251024

REASON 6: BREASTFED BABIES NEED FEWER DOCTOR VISITS

Ball, T. M. and A. L. Wright, "Health Care Costs of Formula-feeding in the First Year of Life," *Pediatrics*, 1999; 103: 870-876.

Fallat, M.D. et al, "Breastfeeding Reduces Incidence of Hospital Admission for Infections in Infants," *Pediatrics*, 1980, 65:1121-24.

Kannaaneh, H., "The Relationship of Bottle Feeding to Malnutrition and Gastroenteritis in a Preindustrial Setting," *Journal of Tropical Pediatrics*, 18:302, 1972.

REASON 7: BREASTMILK FEEDS THE BRAIN…AND LINKS TO INCREASED INTELLIGENCE

NICHD publications, as well as information about the Institute, are available from the NICHD website, http://www.nichd.nih.gov, or from the NICHD Information Resource Center, 1-800-370-2943; E-mail NICHDInformationResourceCenter@mail.nih.gov.

B. Taylor and J. Wadsworth, "Breastfeeding and Child Development at Five Years," *Dev. Med. Child Neurol.*, 26: 73, 1984.

Horwood and Fergusson, "Breastfeeding and Later Cognitive and Academic Outcomes," *Pediatrics*, Jan. 1998.

Lucas, A., "Breast Milk and Subsequent Intelligence Quotient in Children Born Preterm," *Lancet*, 1992, 339:261-262.

Morrow-Tlucak, M., R.H. Haude and C.B. Ernhart, "Breastfeeding and Cognitive Development in the First 2 Years of Life." *Soc Sci Med*, 1988:26; 635-639.

Wang, Y.S. and S.Y. Wu. "The Effect of Exclusive Breastfeeding on Development And Incidence of Infection in Infants." *Journal of Human Lactation*, 1996, 12:27-30.

REFERENCES

REASON 8: PHYSICAL/EMOTIONAL BONDING BETWEEN MOTHER AND CHILD IS INCREASED BY BREASTFEEDING

Acheson, L., "Family violence and Breastfeeding," *Archives of Family Medicine*, 1995, vol. 4, 650-52.

Caplan, M., *To Touch is to Live: The Need for Genuine Affection in an Impersonal World*, Prescott, Arizona: Hohm Press, 2002.

Feldman, R. et al, "Comparison of Skin-to-Skin (Kangaroo) and Traditional Care: Parenting Outcomes and Preterm Infant Development: *Pediatrics,* Vol. 110 No. 1 July 2002, pp. 16-26

Heller, Sharon, *The Vital Touch: How Intimate Contact With Your Baby Leads to Happier, Healthier Development*, New York: Owl Books, 1997.

Klaus, M, and J. Kennell, *Parent-Infant Bonding*, St. Louis: Mosley, 1982.

Ludington, S., *Kangaroo Care: The Best Thing You Can Do to Help Your Preterm Infant*, New York: Bantam, 1993.

Montagu, Ashley, *Touching: The Human Significance of the Skin*, New York: Harper-Collins, 1983.

Sears, James, et al., *Everything You Need to Know About Your Baby from Birth to Age Two* (revised and updated edition), New York: Little, Brown and Company, 2003.

REASON 9: BREASTFED BABIES HAVE LESS NEED TO CRY

Hunziker, U. and R. Barr, *Pediatrics*, 1986, 77, 641-648, "Increased Carrying Reduces Infant Crying: A Randomized Controlled Trial." The researchers discovered that babies at six weeks of age who were carried three or more hours each day (rather than put in an infant seat or crib) were crying 43 percent less than the other infants, particularly in the evening. This study went on to note similar improvements in infant behavior at 4, 8 and 12 weeks.

Michelsson, K., and Christensson, K., et al., "Crying in separated and non-separated newborns: sound spectrographic analysis," *Acta Paediatr.*, 85: 471, 1996.

REASON 10: BREASTFEEDING ENCOURAGES STRESS REDUCTION IN BABY AND MOM

Hunziker, U. and R. Barr, *Pediatrics*, 1986, 77, 641-648, "Increased Carrying Reduces Infant Crying: A Randomized Controlled Trial."

Sears, W. and M. Sears, *The Breastfeeding Book*, Little, Brown & Co., 2000.

REASON 11: BREASTFEEDING IS MUCH LESS COSTLY THAN BOTTLE-FORMULA FEEDING

BottMontgomery, D., and P. Splett, "Economic Benefit of Breast-Feeding Infants Enrolled in WIC," *Journal of the American Dietetic Association* 97:379-385, 1997. PubMed; PMID 9120189

Tuttle, C.R., and K.G. Dewey, "Potential Cost Savings for Medi-Cal, AFDC, Food Stamps, and WIC Programs Associated with Increasing Breast-Feeding among Low-Income Hmong Women in California," *Journal of the American Dietetic Association* 6:885-890, 1996. PubMed; PMID 8784333

REASON 12: BREASTFEEDING BUILDS STRAIGHTER TEETH AND STONGER TEETH

Lesperance, L.M. (M.D., Ph.D.) and H. H. Bernstein (D.O.), Harvard Medical School, *News Review of Harvard Medical School*, Nov. 23, 2004, *see:* http://www.intelihealth.com/IH/ihtIH/WSIHW000/24479/36146/404718.html?d=dmtContent)

Loesche, W.J., "Nutrition and Dental Decay in Infants." *American Journal of Clinical Nutrition,* 41; 423-435, 1985

REASON 13: BREASTFEEDING IS GOOD FOR THE EARTH

See: http://www.ecomall.com/greenshopping/mbr.htm

REASON 14: BREASTFEEDING HELPS MOTHER'S BODY READJUST AFTER PREGNANCY

Chua, S., S. Arulkumaran and I. Lim, et al. "Influence of Breastfeeding and Nipple Stimulation on Postpartum Uterine Activity." *British Journal of Obstetrics and Gynecology* 101:804-805, 1994. PubMed; PMID 7947531

Dewey, K.G., M.J. Heinig and L.A Nommsen, "Maternal Weight-Loss Patterns during Prolonged Lactation." *American Journal of Clinical Nutrition* 58:162-166, 1993. PubMed; PMID 8338042

Subcommittee on Nutrition During Lactation, Committee on Nutritional Status during Pregnancy and Lactation, Food and Nutrition board, Institute of Medicine, National Academy of Science: *Nutrition During Lactation*, Washington, D.C.: National Academy Press, 1991.

REASON 15: BREASTFEEDING ALSO PROTECTS A MOTHER'S HEALTH…THROUGHOUT HER LIFE

Chantry, C.J., P. Auinger, and R. S. Byrd, "Lactation Among Adolescent Mothers and Subsequent Bone and Mineral Density," *Archives of Pediatrics and Adolescent Medicine*, 2004, 158: 650-656.

Gwinn, M.L., "Pregnancy, Breastfeeding and Oral Contraceptives and the Risk of Epithelial Ovarian Cancer." *J. Clin. Epidemiol.* 1990; 43:559-568.

Havard, A.,"Breastfeeding - a cure for endometriosis," *Allaiter ajourd'hui, Quarterly Bulletin of LLL France*, No. 25, Oct. - Dec. 1995.

Karlson, E. and H. Wilson, *Arthritis and Rheumatism*, November 2004; vol. 50: 3458-3467.

Melton, L.J., S.C. Bryant and H.W. Wahner, et al., "Influence of Breastfeeding and Other Reproductive Factors on Bone Mass Later in Life." *Osteoporosis International* 3:76-83, 1993. PubMed; PMID 8453194

Newcomb, P.A., B.E. Storer, and M.P. Longnecker, et al. "Lactation and a Reduced Risk of Premenopausal Breast Cancer." *New England Journal of Medicine* 330:81-87, 1994. PubMed; PMID 8259187

Rosenblatt K.A., and D.B. Thomas, "Lactation and the Risk of Epithelial Ovarian Cancer," *International Journal of Epidemiology*, 1993; 22: 192-197.

Schneider, A.P., "Risk Factors for Ovarian Cancer," *New England Journal of Medicine*, 1987.

Rosenblatt, K.A., et al., "Prolonged Lactation and Endometrial Cancer," *International Journal of Epidemiology*, 1995; 24:499-503

Zheng, T., et al., "Lactation Reduces Breast Cancer Risk in Shandong Province, China," *American Journal of Epidemiology*, 2000, 152 (12): 1129-35.

REASON 16: BREASTFEEDING BUILDS A WOMAN'S SELF-CONFIDENCE

Gussler, J.D, and C.A. Bryant, editors, "Helping Mothers to Breastfeed: Program Strategies for Minority Communities." Lexington, Kentucky, 1984. Nutrition and Health Education Division, Lexington-Fayette County Health Department.

REASON 17: BREASTFEEDING HONORS A WOMAN'S BODY

Yalom, M., *A History of the Breast*. New York: Knopf, 1997.

REASON 18: BREASTFEEDING MAKES TRAVEL EASIER

Dunham, C., et. al., *Mamatoto: A Celebration of Birth*, London: Virago Press, 1991.

REASON 19: BREASTFED BABIES SMELL BETTER

See: http://www.askdrsears.com/html/2/T020400.asp

Heacock, H.J., "Influence of Breast vs Formula Milk in Physiologic Gastroesophageal Reflux in Healthy Newborn Infants," *Journal of Pediatric Gastroenterological Nutrition*, 1992 January; 14(1): 41-6.

REASON 20: BREASTFEEDING IS NATURE'S OBVIOUS PLAN

Righard, L., Alade, M.O., "Effect of Delivery Room Routines on Success of First Breastfeeding." *Lancet*, 336:1105, 1990.

PHOTO CREDITS

The photos in this book represent a small sampling of the work of the photographers listed below. Please see *Contact Information* to learn more about their work. The right to reproduce these photographs was granted to the authors and Hohm Press for purposes of this book only. The copyrights to the photos remain with the photographers. No photos in this book may be reproduced under any circumstances without written permission from the photographers.

Cover image: Five nursing mothers: Kathy Hughes, Karen Zirger, Deedee Olsen, Shayla Townsend and Belinda Holmes. Photographer: Denise Punger, MD, FAAFP, IBCLC. Contact information: Coquelet & Punger Family Medicine, P.A., St. Lucie County, Florida; http://denisepunger.tripod.com; denisepunger@hotmail.com

Frontispiece: Grace Schlesinger, age 6 months; Photographer: Donna Goldman/BuzzPictures. Contact information: www.buzzpictures.com/photos; 415-458-3500

Reason 1 photo: Courtesy of LaLeche League International; Photographer: David C. Arendt. Contact information: www.lalecheleague.org

Reason 2 photo: Photographer: Luke Shantz, Tacoma, WA. Contact information: Luke@SummerLandIsland.com

Reason 3 photo: Courtesy of LaLeche League International; Photographer: Kimberly Cavaliero. Contact information: www.lalecheleague.org

Reason 4 photo: Karen Zirger and two children; Photographer: Denise Punger, MD, FAAFP, IBCLC. Contact information: Coquelet & Punger Family Medicine, P.A., St. Lucie County, Florida; http://denisepunger.tripod.com; denisepunger@hotmail.com

Reason 5 photo: Special thanks to Mandy Denver (photographer) from the Toiyabe Indian Health Project, WIC Program and to Heidi Brown for all her efforts on behalf of this book. Contact information: Heidi Brown, Toiyabe WIC, 52 Tu Su Lane, Bishop, CA 93514

Reason 6 photo: New life Photography by Lesley Mason; Birth Portraiture and Stock photography. Contact information: 313-295-8427; www.newlifephto.net

Reason 7 photo: Photographer: Marilyn Nolt. Contact information: noltphotos@mail.com

Reason 8 photo: Natasha starting to nurse shortly after birth; Franziska Heinze Photography * Doula Services (CD) DONA. Contact information: www.franziskaheinze.com

Reason 9 photo: Breastfeeding in love – Carmen and Lucia. Photographer: Shawna Wentz: Pregnancy, Birth, Breastfeeding and Bonding Photography. Contact information: shawnaw@mothering.com

Reason 10 photo: Dora Locklear with son, Joseph Locklear; Photographer: Denise Punger, MD, FAAFP, IBCLC. Contact information: Coquelet & Punger Family Medicine, P.A., St. Lucie County, Florida; http://denisepunger.tripod.com; denisepunger@hotmail.com

Reason 11 photo: Photographer: Marilyn Nolt. Contact information: noltphotos@mail.com

Reason 12 photo: Photographer: Luke Shantz, Tacoma, WA. Contact information: Luke@SummerLandIsland.com

Reason 13 photo: Mother breastfeeding with dog beside her. Photographer: Kathryn Langsford; Contact information: www.photosbykathryn.com

Reason 14 photo: Belinda Holmes and son; Photographer: Denise Punger, MD, FAAFP, IBCLC. Contact information: Coquelet & Punger Family Medicine, P.A., St. Lucie County, Florida; http://denisepunger.tripod.com; denisepunger@hotmail.com

Reason 15 photo: Dr. Rachel Eitches and twin girls. Photographer: Lloyd Wolf. Contact information: www.lloydwolf.com

Reason 16 photo: Debbie Marin nursing her adopted daughter Munirah Marin. Photographer: TeaJay Piersall. Contact information: teajay@teajayphoto.com

Reason 17 photo: New life Photography by Lesley Mason; Birth Portraiture and Stock photography. Contact information: 313-295-8427; www.newlifephto.net

Reason 18 photo: Photographer: Marilyn Nolt. Contact information: noltphotos@mail.com

OTHER TITLES OF INTEREST FROM HOHM PRESS

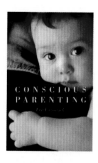

CONSCIOUS PARENTING
By Lee Lozowick

The message of this book is that the first two years are the most crucial time in a child's education and development, and children learn to be healthy and "whole" by living with healthy, whole adults. Offers practical guidance and help for anyone who wishes to bring greater consciousness to every aspect of childraising, including: * conception, pregnancy and birth * emotional development * language usage * role modeling: the mother's role, the father's role * the exposure to various influences * establishing workable boundaries * the choices we make on behalf on our children's education ... and much more.

Paper, 378 pages, $17.95

ISBN: 0-934252-67-X

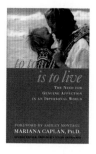

TO TOUCH IS TO LIVE
The Need for Genuine Affection in an Impersonal World
By Mariana Caplan
Foreword by Ashley Montagu

The vastly impersonal nature of contemporary culture, supported by massive child abuse and neglect, and reinforced by growing techno-fascination are robbing us of our humanity. The author takes issue with the trends of the day that are mostly overlooked as being "progressive" or harmless, showing how these trends are actually undermining genuine affection and love. This uncompromising and inspiring work offers positive solutions for countering the effects of the growing depersonalization of our times.

"An important book that brings to the forefront the fundamentals of a healthy world. We must all touch more."

– **Patch Adams, M.D.**

Paper, 272 pages, $19.95

ISBN: 1-890772-24-0

To Order: 800-381-2700, or visit our website, www.hohmpress.com • **Special discounts for bulk orders.**

OTHER TITLES OF INTEREST FROM HOHM PRESS

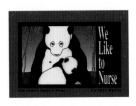

WE LIKE TO NURSE
By Chia Martin
Illustrations by Shukyo Lin Rainey

Research has documented that the advantages of breastfeeding far outweigh the disadvantages in the overall health of the child. This unique children's picture book supports that practice, as it honors the mother-child relationship, reminding young children and mothers alike of their deep feelings for the bond created by nursing. Captivating and colorful illustrations present mother animals nursing their young. The text is simple and warmly encouraging.

"A delightful way to remind the very young of our species' natural heritage as well as our deep kinship with other mammals." – **Jean Liedloff, author** *Continuum Concept.*

Paper, 36 pages, 16 full-color illustrations, $9.95   ISBN: 0-934252-45-9

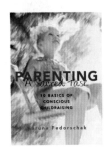

PARENTING, A SACRED TASK
10 Basics of Conscious Childraising
by Karuna Fedorschak

Moving beyond our own self-centered focus and into the realm of generosity and expansive love is the core of spiritual practice. This book can help us to make that move. It highlights 10 basic elements that every parent can use to meet the everyday demands of childraising. Turning that natural duty into a sacred task is what this book is about. Topics include: love, attention, boundaries, food, touch, help and humor.

"There is no more rigorous path to spiritual development than that of being a parent. Thank you to Karuna Fedorschak for remind us that parenting is a sacred task." – **Peggy O'Mara, Editor and Publisher,** *Mothering Magazine.*

Paper, 158 pages, $12.95   ISBN: 1-890772-30-5

To Order: 800-381-2700, or visit our website, www.hohmpress.com • **Special discounts for bulk orders.**